TABLE OF CONTENTS

CANNABIS TINCTURE RECIPES ANYONE CAN MAKE 67

INTRODUCTION

Cannabis is an impressively versatile plant, taking on a wide range of forms to offer the ultimate in variety. One such form is a cannabis tincture, a type of cannabis-infused product with a long and storied history that dates back generations. Convenient, user-friendly, and smoke-free, tinctures offer a fuss-free option that appeals to new and seasoned consumers alike.

A tincture is a liquid product, formulated with a high-percentage alcohol and presented in handy dropper-top bottles. Essentially, a tincture is a cannabis-infused alcohol, created using a precise process.

Similar to the process of extracting cannabis oil, a tincture utilizes a solvent (alcohol) to extract cannabinoids (THC and CBD) and terpenes from the cannabis plant. Alcohol is both the solvent and an ingredient in the final product, which is where tinctures differ from traditional cannabis oils.

Interestingly, tinctures were the primary form of cannabis-based medicine for decades, up until the United States outlawed cannabis. Now, as a growing number of states legalize medicinal and/or recreational cannabis consumption, tinctures have made an impressive comeback.

Although some individuals make DIY tinctures at home, most consumers prefer the convenience and consistency of professionally-formulated tinctures instead. The process of making a homemade cannabis tincture can be a hassle, while purchasing high-quality options from your favorite dispensary delivers a far more enjoyable and reliably excellent experience.

CBD OIL TINCTURE FOR BEGINNERS

You've probably seen the very cool apothecary-style amber bottle that holds the oil tincture and wondered how you're supposed to use it, right? You skip over it because it's a new product and you're not sure what to do with it.

Let's talk about why you should give this high-quality full-spectrum hemp oil a shot.

What Is CBD oil Tincture?

CBD oil tinctures are not the same as CBD oil; tinctures are alcohol-based and the other is oil-based – both will aid in treating various medical conditions but are consumed in different ways.

CBD oil can be infused in gummies, brownies, chocolate or it can be used with a vape pen or as a topical balm, just to name a few ways that make CBD oil different than CBD tinctures.

If this is your first time considering expanding your curiosity into other CBD products besides topicals and edibles, you're in the right place!

First, let's discuss the difference between the hemp plant and the marijuana plant.

The hemp plant is only part of the cannabis Sativa family while the marijuana plant is from either the cannabis Sativa family of the cannabis Indica family.

Hemp is thinner and glossier while marijuana is bushier with fuller leaves.

What are the CBD Benefits?

CBD tinctures are made from high CBD – low THC hemp so it won't make you stoned. You will, however, receive all the wonderful benefits this delectable elixir has to offer like its

• Anti-inflammatory properties

• Anxiety relief

• And insomnia, to name a few.

How to Use CBD Oil for Beginners

There are many ways of consuming CBD tinctures. One way of including this into your diet is by adding it to coffee, tea, soup or any other food you'd like.

The effects won't be instant but you'll still get the benefits.

You could also use the dropper but before you go ham and use a full dropper try taking a few drops at a time to see what the best dosage is for you.

CBD tinctures are labeled to help you understand the potency of the tincture. Use this to help you determine what's best for you.

Keep a record of the dosages you take. Monitor how you feel and adjust accordingly.

If you don't feel much, you've probably taken too little.

If you knock out, you've probably taken too much.

Start with one to two drops and see how you feel before you up the dosage.

Fortunately, there are no serious side effects when you consume CBD tinctures.

You might get drowsy or cottonmouth but nothing that is alarming.

Some people won't consider drowsiness as a side effect if you're in need of some serious Zs. Glass half full? I think so.

If you decide to take it straight from the bottle make sure you take it sublingually (under the tongue) and hold it there for a minute.

This is the optimum way of taking it as it'll absorb quickly into the bloodstream.

Countless anecdotal evidence is out there that proves CBD is helpful in relieving many ailments that prevent people from living in comfort. Tinctures are fast-acting and effective.

Patients Claimed They've Received CBD Relief From:

• Seizures

• Chronic pain

• Cancer cell growth

• Diabetes

• Nausea

• ADHD and more

Because there aren't enough studies out there on CBD tinctures these statements have not been evaluated by the food and drug administration.

It's a shame that there aren't enough "official" studies out there to make this medicine accessible to more people without the fear of repercussions associated with using the medicinal properties of this solution.

Taking CBD oil tincture for beginners won't prevent any diseases but it'll sure make life a little brighter and more comfortable if you're experiencing pain or depression.

CBD tinctures can come in different potencies so if you're just starting to dabble in this product you can begin by trying a 300mg hemp oil tincture, or if that's not strong enough you can check out the CBD hemp oil tincture 900mg, and last but not least, if you're a bold soul that needs something that's going to pack a punch because you have some serious ailment that requires the big guns try the 1800 mg CBD oil tincture.

This is also great if you're a gym rat that goes heavy on the weight lifting and need something for that post-workout muscle soreness that kicks you right in the gut the next day, thank you DOMS!

Tinctures are easy and convenient to carry around in your gym bag or backpack for easy access so you can manage your pain effectively.

If you decide to use the extra potent CBD hemp oil 1800 mg make sure you reach out to customer service to see if it's right for you.

CBD tinctures are great for beginners because of its discreet way of consuming the benefits of CBD oil for beginners without smoking the traditional joint or blunt.

So if your curiosity has peeked and you have an illness that needs attention without going the pharmaceutical route, tinctures are the way to go to

• Reduce pain and inflammation

• Relieve muscle spasm

• Calm your nerves

• Reduce stress

• Help with artery blockage

• Get a restful night's sleep

• Help you focus

• Manage cancer symptoms

• Reduce seizures

• And more

So don't hesitate to explore this high-quality product that's lab-tested to ensure it's premium ingredients are consistent and safe.

Instructions for extracting CBD oil at home

Only certain strains of cannabis offer the best-quality CBD. If you are growing your own, you should know that some strains have a high content of THC and CBD as well. Two good examples of high CBD/low THC strains are Avi-dekel and industrial hemp.

Find a strain of plant with a high CBD and low THC level. As you prepare, you will need to ensure that you have a well-ventilated area. You should also have a solid understanding of how much CBD oil you would like to have in each treat and calculate this ahead of time.

To extract the oil, you will need a cup of carrier oil (virgin coconut oil is great) and 14 g of the right type of CBD buds.

CBD Extraction Instructions:

• Grind the entire hemp plant, and put it in a canning jar with the carrier oil, placing the lid on tightly.

• Put the jar and a washrag in a saucepan with a few inches of water, and bring it to just below boiling, leaving it there for 3 hours and replacing water if it evaporates.

- Using tongs or oven mitts, give the jar a shake about every half an hour.

- When 3 hours are up, turn off the burner, and cover the pot with a towel.

- Allow the jar to cool for 3 hours, then repeat the process, leaving the jar in the pot with the towel on it overnight.

- Repeat the process over the course of a few days for stronger oil.

- When you have your oil, you can strain it through a cheesecloth.

If you are using CBD oil to cook, you should note that the boiling point is a maximum of 180 degrees C. These types of oils are sensitive to light and heat, so you should store them in a dark glass bottle and in a cool area.

What are CBD tinctures?

A CBD tincture is a liquid extract of the cannabis plant, that is taken orally as an herbal preparation to relieve chronic pain, balance mood and assist with sleep. CBD tincture contains cannabidiol (CBD), along with a host of other active constituents of the cannabis plant, such as cannabinoids, alkaloids, glycosides, minerals, phytonutrients and terpenes.

Cannabis tincture is an alcohol-based concentrate, or simply put, it is weed infused with alcohol.

All of the cannabinoids and terpenes are removed from the rest of the plant and mixed in with the alcohol.

This solvent is frequently used for cannabis extraction, because it does a great job of separating the active substances from the rest of the plant material.

Tinctures are usually odorless, discreet and great for carrying around.

Cannabis tinctures have been used for centuries for medicinal purposes and were the most commonly used form of cannabis prior to the 1930's US cannabis prohibition, which subsequently resulted in a worldwide illegalization of this plant.

It's hard to imagine that less than a century ago cannabis tinctures were listed in the US Pharmacopeia, and were used throughout the country as a completely legitimate way for treating numerous conditions.

CBD tinctures are most commonly made from the industrial hemp plant, a strain of cannabis that has been bred to contain less than 0.3% THC. However, CBD tinctures can also be made from low-THC strains of the marijuana plant.

For many who suffer from chronic pain, tinctures are a preferred method of CBD ingestion because of the ease of use, long shelf life and speed of delivery. CBD tinctures are administered sublingually, by taking a small dose of the extract under the tongue. The CBD is absorbed promptly by the mucous membrane in the mouth into the bloodstream, delivering relief within 15 minutes.

CBD tinctures are easy to make at home—you won't need a chemistry degree to make your own.

HOMEMADE VERSUS COMMERCIAL

What is a commercial CBD tincture?

A commercial CBD tincture is an herbal cannabis preparation that is manufactured by a commercial producer for public sale. Commercial CBD tinctures commonly contain CBD oil extracted from the hemp or marijuana plant via commercial extraction methods and must comply with strict standards for quality, efficacy, purity, and labeling.

What is a homemade CBD tincture?

A homemade CBD tincture is a CBD-infused herbal preparation that you can make yourself at home by dissolving plant material—such as the flower, leaves and stem of the hemp plant—into a liquid solvent, such as high-proof alcohol, or a non-alcoholic carrier liquid, such as coconut oil, olive oil or vegetable glycerine.

What are the differences between commercial and homemade?

When it comes to choosing between homemade versus commercial CBD oil tinctures, it is essential to note which route works better for your lifestyle. Commercial products offer convenience and purity, while DIY tinctures provide full control over potency and ingredients.

Purity

The significant difference between homemade versus commercial is purity. A commercial CBD oil tincture is more thoroughly filtered than a homemade concoction. Commercial producers are required to meet strict standards for purity and utilize sophisticated filtration processes to thoroughly remove solvent and contaminants from the cannabis extract.

Ingredients

With a homemade CBD tincture, you have the freedom to select the type of cannabis you wish to extract your CBD from—if you'd prefer to avoid THC, you can use industrial hemp. If you're in a legal state and aren't averse to the effects of THC, then you can make your extract from a high-CBD strain of marijuana.

You also have the choice of liquids to extract your CBD into. If you wish to go the traditional route, then you can select a quality, high-proof alcohol. If you are sensitive to alcohol and would prefer a non-alcoholic tincture, then you can make your CBD tincture using vegetable oil or vegetable glycerine as the solvent.

Potency

While it's easy and convenient to purchase a CBD tincture online or from a store, making your own CBD tincture at home allows you to have full control over the concentration of CBD. By tweaking the amount of plant matter, or experimenting with different strains of cannabis, you can create your own signature CBD tincture with a potency that's perfect for you.

A Primer on CBD and the Endocannabinoid System

All humans have endocannabinoid systems. The endocannabinoid system is a complex network of receptors and neurotransmitters whose role is to maintain the chemical stability in the body, also known as homeostasis.

Whenever this stability is compromised, the endocannabinoid system produces its natural endocannabinoids to bring the homeostasis back. Sometimes, though, the system cannot release enough endocannabinoids to solve chemical imbalances.

And since the endocannabinoid system controls the vast majority of biological processes — from memory to temperature control to pain perception and immune function — the deficiencies in endocannabinoid production has been linked by scientists to a wide range of physiological and mental illnesses.

This is where CBD starts to shine.

THC vs. CBD Tinctures

Before you purchase your tincture, you should know what's available to you and what will work best. The three most common forms of cannabis tincture contain THC, CBD or various combinations of the two in ratios like 1:1.

CBD is said to have many of the same health benefits as THC without any of the mind-altering effects. With research on CBD and hemp illustrating it's merit, recent laws have made it easier to produce and sell CBD products with less than .3% THC in the United States. As a result, CBD doesn't face the same legal obstacles as THC and can be sold nationwide.

On the other hand, any tinctures containing more than .3% THC can only be legally purchased in states with legalized cannabis.

Is a CBD Tincture the Same as CBD Oil?

Some people seem to have difficulty separating CBD tincture from CBD oil, and the fact that both have similar preparation and packaging doesn't help matters. Well, the distinction can be seen in their elements.

While CBD oils are prepared by infusing hemp extracts in carrier oils like coconut oil and MCT oil, CBD tinctures are made by dissolving hemp extracts in alcohol-based solvents. CBD tinctures make for a higher bioavailability, have a long shelf life, and the dosage varies.

CBD oils usually have a nutty/earthy flavor, and some people are not fond of that taste, but CBD tinctures are infused with artificial terpenes and flavors, making them more palatable, especially for beginners.

But CBD tinctures are not just for new CBD users. Experienced users favor CBD tinctures too because of their flexibility as far as the ingestion.

How Do I Use a CBD Tincture?

CBD tinctures typically come with a dropper or oral syringe, and if you are a new CBD user, begin with small doses.

An overdose may not result in any negative consequences, but to get the best results, start with a small dose and adjust your intake depending on how your body reacts.

The following are some of the ways you may use a CBD tincture:

Sublingual Ingestion

Research shows that sublingual CBD ingestion causes the most powerful effects. First off, shake the bottle well to ensure the contents are mixed properly, and that there's enough CBD in each serving.

Using a dropper or an oral syringe, administer the recommended amount of CBD underneath your tongue, and hold for 60 – 90 seconds before you swallow. You may consume it once or twice a day.

Ensure that you buy a flavored CBD tincture so that you don't develop a hesitation toward consuming CBD regularly.

Holding the tincture under your tongue for at least a minute enhances absorption through the sublingual artery, and the CBD is first carried to your heart, and then to your brain.

Food and Beverages

Maybe you are not fond of how CBD tinctures taste like, regardless of whether or not they are flavored, and you can get around this by consuming them along with your food or drink.

Whether sitting before you is a bowl of soup or salad, a cup of coffee or tea, or a plate of rice, you can infuse them with the tincture. But note that this method lessens the impact of CBD, though.

On the upside, this method makes consuming CBD fun.

Why Can't I Vape CBD Tinctures?

CBD tinctures are hemp extracts dissolved in alcohol, and they are designed for traditional ingestion, not vaping.

Unless the manufacturer states that you can vape it, avoid vaping CBD tinctures because it can affect your health.

You see, cannabinoids interact very well with body cells, but the base oils used in CBD tinctures have been found to cling onto the lung surface, thus attracting bacteria and increasing vulnerability to lipoid pneumonia.

The alcohol in CBD tinctures enhances the absorption of CBD, and so, CBD tinctures are best ingested via the mouth, and not to be smoked or vaped.

Health Dangers Of Vaping Cannabis Oil

• A Health Danger. Vaping cannabis or any substance for that matter is contraindicated for anyone, especially those with asthma or respiratory conditions.

• May Cause Long Term Damage

• Potentially More Toxic. Additional ingredients added to vape oil cartridges, like the popular thinning agent propylene glycol, become carcinogenic when heated. Avoid any product that contains propylene glycol (PG), vegetable glycerine (VG), MCT coconut oil (MCT), and/or vitamin E acetate.

• Enticing to Minors. Vaping nicotine has become a trend with underage youth, and vaping CBD may follow suit due to its easy accessibility.

How Do CBD Tinctures Compare to Prescription Drugs?

Research shows that CBD is effective at eliminating various health problems, but the big question is; how does CBD stack up against conventional medicine?

Does CBD do a better job of treating certain ailments than conventional medicine? And if this is the case, are people turning away from OTC drugs in favor of CBD?

CBD might be effective at treating certain health conditions, but this is not to mean that it should take the place of conventional medicine. For the best results, both treatments should be used jointly.

Whether you are preparing for a speech and anxiety is getting the best of you, or you can't seem to fall (and stay) asleep or are looking to relax after an intense workout, CBD can be most helpful.

But there's an ocean of other health problems that CBD cannot resolve, and it was best to use conventional medicine.

What's the Difference Between Strong Tinctures and Weak Tinctures?

Tinctures with high CBD concentration cost more than tinctures with low CBD concentration, but consumers wonder precisely how the differences in CBD concentration affect results.

It's hard to come up with a standard explanation because different people react differently to CBD concentrations; some people respond best to low CBD concentrations, while others respond best to high CBD concentrations.

But then again, if a CBD tincture contains less than 50mgs CBD per milliliter, that's a very weak concentration, and the results may be stunted.

People who are new to CBD usually start with weaker concentrations and work their way up.

Can CBD Tinctures Get Me Drunk?

CBD tinctures may contain alcohol, but it is not enough alcohol to get you drunk... well, unless you consume an inordinately large amount of CBD tinctures.

CBD tinctures can be either broad-spectrum or full-spectrum, and some of the additional compounds include CBN, CBG, and terpenes.

The appropriate dosage for you depends on three main factors: your age, your health status, and the medication you are on. If you have a high tolerance for CBD, you might have to ingest a little bit more.

How Much Tincture

Generally speaking, there's no ideal serving of CBD tinctures per se. The proper CBD oil tincture serving size solely depends on the preferences and needs of an individual. There is a suggested starting size, and you are encouraged to start "low and slow" as a beginner. CBD has a different effect on everyone, ranging from the optimal dosage needed to the after-effects/side effects. Some people are not able to process CBD, and these are people who don't understand the effects or don't feel the effects of CBD. What's more, CBD tinctures come in a variety of concentrations and sizes. So it's not a one-shoe-fits-all situation when it comes to using tinctures. Some of the factors involved include:

• The body weight of an individual

• The CBD sensitivity of an individual

• The CBD concentration

• The magnitude of one's condition

When these factors are considered, there will be some trial and error when determining the proper serving to ingest. If you are a first time user, it's advisable that you begin low and slowly grow your serving. The liquid solution is measured in fluid ounces (oz.) or milliliters (mL) and CBD content labeled milligrams. But all in all, when it comes down to it, the hemp oil tincture you ingest daily is up to you. We recommend not taking more than 100mg per day, and be consistent and take it daily.

When it's gone, you will know if you miss it or not.

Here are a suggested daily dosage beginning points:

Mild

85-149 lbs. (10mg)

150-229 lbs. (15mg)

230+ lbs. (25mg)

Moderate

85-149 lbs. (15mg)

150-229 lbs. (20mg)

230+ lbs. (30mg)

Strong

85-149 lbs. (20mg)

150-229 lbs. (30mg)

230+ lbs. (40mg)

So what time should I take my CBD Tincture? If you are a beginner at using CBD tinctures, it's recommended that you consume it at night. CBD generally provides a calm feeling that will make you feel relaxed and potentially sleepy. Wind down your day with a CBD tincture. Just start with small quantities and steadily increase the amount. You can take a small amount in the morning and another one at night before sleeping. But as always, consult with your medical practitioner first before embarking on a CBD regimen — especially if you are on ANY medication already.

How Does CBD Tincture Affect the Body?

Before we look at what happens when you ingest CBD or use it topically, we need to examine how the body's endocannabinoid system functions. In the brain, you'll find a network of CB1 receptors. These receptors are associated with essential brain functions such as pain, movement, coordination, and emotions. Elsewhere – such as the tonsils, spleen, and parts of the immune system – you'll find CB2 receptors.

Research on the extract is still in its early stages. Cannabinoids such as CBD may activate these receptors. As a result, they could help enhance related functions and therefore improve your health and boost your mood.

How Long Will It Take to Feel the Effects of CBD?

Depending on the dosage, it can take up to 30 minutes to feel the effects of CBD. As there is no psychoactive ingredient in CBD tincture, you won't feel "high." Instead, you will notice a calming sensation or a reduction in pain.

Is CBD Tincture Legal?

Since CBD is non-psychotropic and won't get you high, it is legal in most places. Of course, it's always best to check your local laws. Generally, if your CBD tincture is made with hemp (which contains little-to-no THC), you shouldn't have a problem. According to the World Health Organization (WHO), CBD is not addictive, and is generally safe and well-tolerated.

METHODS OF MAKING CBD TINCTURES

Making your own CBD tinctures at home is pretty easy, but before you get started, you'll need to decide on the method that's right for you.

The first thing to consider when deciding on your preferred method is the solvent.

Solvents

• Alcohol

Traditionally, herbal tinctures are made with alcohol. Using alcohol as the solvent produces a potent CBD extract that is very quickly absorbed by the body when taken sublingually (under the tongue).

While the amount of alcohol you will consume when taking an alcohol-based CBD tincture is minimal, it still needs to be metabolized by the body. If you have a sensitivity to alcohol, or you dislike the flavor or mouthfeel of alcohol, you should consider non-alcoholic methods for making CBD tincture.

• Vegetable oil

If you'd prefer to use a non-alcoholic base for your tincture, or find high-grade alcohol hard to source, then vegetable oil method is a popular alternative. This method is simple and accessible, as it uses ingredients that you're likely to already have in your pantry, such as coconut, olive or sunflower oil.

CBD tinctures made from vegetable oil are ideal to add to food and drink. If you're interested in making your own CBD edibles, then the vegetable oil method may be the best match for you.

• Glycerine

Vegetable glycerin is a clear liquid commonly derived from soy, palm and coconuts. Its lipid structure makes it an ideal solvent to replace alcohol because the cannabinoids attach to the lipids during extraction.

Keep in mind that CBD tinctures made with vegetable glycerin—also known as glycerites— tend to be lower in potency than alcohol-based CBD tinctures, but they're a great alternative for people who prefer to avoid alcohol.

Steeping

Steeping describes the process of dissolving the plant extract into the solvent. That may sound complicated, but steeping is a fairly simple and familiar process. If you've ever made a cup of tea, you'll understand that the tea leaves need to steep in water for a period of time for the flavors and tannins of the tea to infuse into the water.

There are two methods of steeping. The first is the traditional method of maceration. The second is the more modern method of percolation.

The decision between maceration and percolation depends on one important factor: time.

Traditional maceration – the slow and simple method

Maceration is the most traditional method of making a tincture and is ideal for beginners. Simply add plant material and solvent to an airtight jar, and leave to steep in a cool, dark place.

You'll require patience with this method, as it takes at least six weeks for the CBD and phytonutrients of the cannabis plant to dissolve into your chosen solvent.

Percolation – the quick but complex method

If you'd prefer to speed up the extraction process, you can use the percolation method. As with maceration, plant matter and solvent are added to an air-tight jar. But instead of leaving your jar on a shelf to steep for a lengthy period, the jar is instead placed into a water bath and brought to simmer.

While percolation is a bit more complex than maceration, and requires some extra utensils, this method is an ideal way to cut down the steeping time if you need your CBD tincture in a hurry.

Ingredients for making your own

Now that you've decided on your preferred solvent and extraction method, it's time to select your ingredients. What ingredients do you need to make one?

The first and most important ingredient that you'll need to make a CBD tincture is cannabis.

• Cannabis

CBD tincture can be made from the flower, leaf and stem of the cannabis plant. It is common to make them from "trim" or "shake," which is the surplus cannabis left over after harvesting the flower. Trim can be used alone or combined with flower as an affordable option.

As noted earlier, CBD tincture can be made from either industrial hemp or high-CBD strains of marijuana, which are different types of Cannabis plants.

• Industrial Hemp

We recommend using industrial hemp for your homemade CBD tincture. This is because industrial hemp contains a high concentration of CBD, and less than 0.3%

THC, so it won't get you high or have any unwanted psychoactive effects.

• Marijuana

If you don't mind the effects of THC, and you're located in a state where cannabis is legal, you may choose to make your homemade CBD tincture from marijuana. We recommend a high-CBD, low-THC strain of marijuana, such as Ringo's Gift, Harlequin, or ACDC. This will limit the effect of the THC, and maximize the effect of CBD, while taking advantage of the 'entourage effect', which describes the synergistic relationship between these two cannabinoids.

• Solvents

The next ingredient you'll need is your solvent. As we discussed earlier, the solvent is the liquid component of your tincture, and is what the CBD is extracted into.

You can choose between alcohol, vegetable oil, or glycerin as your solvent.

i. Alcohol

For alcohol-based tinctures, you'll need a high-proof alcohol that is 60-70% ethyl alcohol or ethanol. Everclear is a recommended source because of its high alcohol content, as is 151 Rum. You want to make sure that you are using food-safe alcohol that is not denatured.

ii. Vegetable Oil

Vegetable oil is probably the easiest solvent to source, as well as the most cost-effective. A wide range of vegetable oils can be purchased from the grocery store—in fact, you may already have the perfect vegetable oil in your pantry, ready to be made into a CBD tincture.

Not all vegetable oils are made equal when it comes to tinctures. Here's what we recommend:

Liquid Coconut Oil: Cannabinoids rely on fatty acids as a binding agent, and since coconut oil is rich in fatty acids, it's an ideal oil for your homemade CBD tincture. For tinctures, it is necessary to purchase liquid coconut oil, as coconut oil becomes solid at room temperature.

Extra Virgin Olive Oil: Olive oil is regarded worldwide as a healthy oil, rich in antioxidants and oleic acid. An added benefit of olive oil is that it is efficient in preserving terpenes from the cannabis plant, providing a whole-plant extract.

Sunflower Oil: Sunflower oil is an affordable option, with a milder flavor than coconut and olive oil. Sunflower Oil is well suited to percolation, as it has good thermal stability. Additionally, sunflower oil is high in lecithin, which helps to increase the shelf life of your tincture.

iii. Glycerin

It's important to note that not all glycerin is appropriate for human consumption. For a glycerin-based CBD tincture, be sure to purchase food-grade vegetable glycerin from a trusted, sustainable source.

Tools and supplies for making CBD tinctures?

What makes it so easy to make CBD tinctures at home is the fact that the tools and supplies required are regular household items.

Here's what you'll need to make a tincture via the traditional maceration method:

• Mason jar

• Cheesecloth or coffee filters

• Glass bottle (amber or cobalt glass works best)

• Baking tray

• Parchment paper

• Timer

If you're making your tincture using the percolator method, you'll also need:

• Glass or metal bowl

• Saucepan

• Candy thermometer

How to decarboxylate your cannabis

Before you start infusing, you'll need to decarb your cannabis. Don't worry—this is a simple step that you can do in your kitchen.

Decarboxylation is the process of heating your cannabis at a specific temperature to activate the cannabinoids. In the case of CBD, decarboxylation (decarbing for short) transforms the inactive CBD-A cannabinoid of raw cannabis into active CBD.

• Preheat your oven to 240°F.

• With your fingers, break your cannabis into small chunks.

• Line a baking tray with parchment paper.

• Distribute the cannabis evenly onto the paper and place the tray into the oven.

• Allow the cannabis to toast for 20 minutes. Gently move the cannabis around with a wooden spoon so that it heats evenly. Put back into the oven.

• When the cannabis starts to look lightly toasted, it's time to take it out of the oven. Hemp and high-CBD strains of marijuana generally take 60-90 minutes to decarb.

• Remove from oven and leave to cool.

Benefits of Using a Cannabis Tincture

Using a cannabis tincture has many advantages compared to consuming other forms of cannabis, and it's no wonder many consumers choose this type of product for cannabis consumption.

• Practical and easy to use – Consuming cannabis tinctures doesn't require any additional devices or preparation in advance (unlike smoking or vaporizing, where you need to prepare a vaping device or roll a joint). You can carry tinctures with you and take them whenever you remember, even if you are in a hurry. They come in a bottle with a dropper, so when you want to take your dose, you can simply place a couple of drops under your tongue. As simple as that.

• Discrete consumption – Many cannabis users are not comfortable with smoking or vaping cannabis in public, especially because of the odor that comes as a result of this way of taking cannabis. On the other hand, cannabis tinctures are odorless, and besides sublingual use, you can consume them by adding a couple of drops into coffee or juice for more discrete consumption.

• The flexibility of use – Cannabis tinctures are an excellent ally in making other cannabis products because they're often the basis for many food recipes and sweets, or added to juices, water, and even bath bombs.

• Fast onset time – As we mentioned earlier, tinctures are mostly used sublingually. When the tincture is applied under the tongue, cannabis quickly gets into the blood through numerous capillaries and vessels in the mouth, and you will feel the effects of it very soon. That's why cannabis tinctures have a quicker onset time than cannabis edibles or capsules, which needs to go through the digestive tract before you can feel the effects of it.

• Fine-tuning dosage – Cannabis tinctures allow consumers to better control their doses since tinctures are applied drop by drop. Consumers can try different dosages until they find the one the works best for them. This is not a case with some other cannabis-based products (e.g.edibles, capsules) that have predetermined dosages of cannabis that can't be changed for every use.

• Slows Down Neurodegeneration

Antioxidants found in CBD tinctures act on the endocannabinoid system and other brain signaling networks to prevent neurodegeneration in brain cells, as research indicates. This slows down cognitive impairments and should be further investigated in terms of preventing neurodegenerative disorders in elderly people.

• A Natural Anti-Inflammatory

CBD has the ability to boost immune function in the body by interacting with CB2 cannabinoid receptors in the immune system, hence its strong anti-inflammatory effects. People often switch to CBD from OTC medications because it reduces inflammation and alleviates pain in a safe and natural way.

• Can Help You Kick the Bad Habits

According to recent research, the use of CBD can help people quit smoking and reduce the withdrawal symptoms caused by substance dependence.

The researchers noted that CBD reduced the severity of different symptoms experienced by patients with substance use disorders, including anxiety, mood swings, hot flashes, pain, and insomnia.

Are There Any Side Effects?

Yes, although they are ridiculously mild compared to many officially acknowledged treatments.

Even the WHO considers cannabidiol an effective and relatively safe substance.

According to studies, doses as high as 1500 mg of CBD taken daily are well tolerated in humans.

So, what can happen when you take too much of your CBD tincture?

1. Dry Mouth

This is a common phenomenon among all cannabis strains and products, whether from hemp or marijuana.

That's because both CBD and THC inhibit the saliva production in your mouth. You can easily deal with it by simply drinking plenty of water or other hydrating liquids prior to, during, and after consuming CBD.

2. Low Blood Pressure

Higher doses of CBD tinctures can cause a small drop in blood pressure. If you have been diagnosed with low pressure or are taking medication for high blood pressure, this may be troublesome because the pressure might drop too low and cause lightheadedness. Most people consider this feeling uncomfortable.

3. Dizziness

Again, at higher doses, CBD can induce drowsiness. Dosages of about 50-100 mg of CBD per session will produce sedative effects. If this is how large amounts of cannabidiol affect you, it's important not to consume CBD tinctures before working on heavy machinery or a driving a vehicle.

4. Negative Interactions With Other Medications

CBD affects the cytochrome P-450 system that is responsible for metabolizing active substances in drugs. It inhibits the system's ability to process certain drugs, which can lead to increased levels of these compounds in your body at one time.

Consequently, you can experience adverse reactions, and sometimes, overdose on those drugs.

If you're on any medications you fear could interact with CBD, it's crucial to consult with your doctor prior to incorporating CBD tinctures into your supplementation plan.

How to Use a Cannabis Tincture?

Cannabis tincture is usually consumed with a dropperful, commonly known as a dropper.

Placing a few drops under your tongue will get you high fast. Thanks to the veins underneath the tongue (part of the arterial system), cannabinoids rapidly enter the bloodstream, creating cerebral effects in a matter of minutes.

With tinctures, it's also very easy to control your high (or the dose of medicinal cannabis). If you sense that you require a bit more, drip a few more drops.

Remember, it's always better to start low and work your way up if needed.

Safety first!

Making tinctures involves the use of high-proof alcohol. All of the stuff we recommend is great for the job, but it's also flammable!

Here are a few steps to make tincture creation as uneventful as possible:

• No open flames – That means no smoking. Even a small spark can be enough to create a massive fire under the right conditions.

- No gas stoves – It's insanely dangerous to attempt cooking tinctures near gas-burner stoves. Alcohol fumes + a gas stove is a recipe for an accidental fire. If your stove uses gas, try using a hot plate if possible, but under no circumstances should you take the chance of using a gas burner stove.

- Ensure Good Ventilation – High-proof alcohol makes fumes that can be easily ignited when they build up. If you keep the area well-ventilated, the concentration of flammable fumes in the air stays low enough that it can't be combusted. In other words, make sure there's new, clean air in your cooking area to avoid a flaming mishap.

- Keep a dry-chemical fire extinguisher handy – As long as you follow the rules above, you'll be fine making your own tinctures. However, it's always a good idea to be prepared! You can get extinguishers at hardware stores or online. Either way, it's a good thing to have around

your house in case of an emergency whether you're

making tinctures or not.

CANNABIS TINCTURE RECIPES ANYONE CAN MAKE

You'll agree that one of the best things about the cannabis industry is the availability of weed in many different, innovative, and healthy forms.

Tinctures are a prime example, as they are a healthy, smokeless way to medicate with cannabis.

And they aren't just a temporary novelty — they've been around for centuries and their popularity is growing because of our awakened love for healthy things.

To help you dive headfirst into this topic, I chose five wonderful tincture recipes that you may want to try making yourself at home..

How to Make a Cannabis Tincture?

Cannabis tinctures can be made either with alcohol, glycerin or coconut oil. There are some great recipes circling around the web.

Creating tinctures usually requires a few weeks, but I chose recipes that are fairly simple to make and don't require that much time. If you own a botanical extractor such as the Magical Butter Machine, even better, because it can make your work much simpler.

First off, a few important tips:

• Depending on what you want to achieve, you can always add more cannabis for a more potent tincture.

• For alcohol extractions: the stronger the alcohol – the stronger the tincture.

• The high from THC-rich tinctures starts very quickly upon consumption, and lasts for about three hours.

• You can make your own CBD tincture by using high-CBD buds instead of high-THC buds.

Green Dragon Recipe (Slow Method)

The process itself is quite easy, but it does take a while, and requires some jar shaking every day.

This type of extraction demands a high-percentage alcohol, because it's the best possible medium for cannabis infusion.

You will need:

• 30 g (about 1 oz) of weed of your choice

• 950 ml (1 qt) of high-proof alcohol (Everclean, or pure grain alcohol)

• Mason jar with a lid

• Grinder

• Glass dropper

• Coffee filters or cheesecloth

Directions:

1. The first thing you need to do is to grind and decarboxylate your buds.

2. Once that's done, place the weed and the alcohol in the jar, close the lid tightly, and store it in a dark cabinet.

3. Shake the contents of the jar on a daily basis (or every other day), and repeat this for at least 2 weeks.

4. Remove the crumbles from the tincture by using a coffee filter (or cheesecloth), until there's no plant material left in the liquid.

5. Pour the tincture in the dropper, and store it in the fridge.

Master Wu's Green Dragon Recipe (Fast Method)

This method is actually an upgraded Green Dragon recipe, very similar to the original but much faster.

For this one you'll need:

• 30 g (about 1 oz) of weed of your choice

• 950 ml (1 qt) of high-proof alcohol (Everclean, or pure grain alcohol)

• Mason jar with a lid

• Deep cooking pot

• Grinder

• Glass dropper

• Coffee filters or cheesecloth

Directions:

1. The start is exactly the same as with the original recipe. Finely grind your buds, decarb them, combine the weed and alcohol in a jar, and close the lid tightly.

This is where things get different:

2. "Cook" the cannabis/alcohol jar in a deep pot filled with water for 20 minutes, keeping the temperature at 170°C.

3. Filter out the plant material from the mixture, pour it into smaller glass containers or droppers, and your cannabis tincture is ready for use!

Weed Tincture (Cold Method)

For this one you will need very similar ingredients:

- 30 g (about 1 oz) of weed of your choice

- 950 ml (1 qt) of high-proof alcohol (Everclean, or pure grain alcohol)

- Mason jar with a lid

- Grinder

- Glass dropper

- Coffee filters or cheesecloth

Directions:

1. The first few steps are the same: Grind, decarboxylate, mix the weed with the alcohol in your mason jar, and close it tightly.

2. The following step differs. Place the jar in a freezer for five days, and shake the contents once a day.

3. You don't need to worry about the jar breaking from the low-temperature liquid expansion, because alcohol has a much lower freezing point compared to water.

4. Purify the mixture with coffee filters or cheesecloths, and store it in a dropper or any other glass container.

The Ed Rosenthal Method

I'm a fan of Ed Rosenthal. He seems to come up with original (or least original to me) ways of doing things, but even better, he always has a reason behind his methods.

Supplies:

• Weed

• High-Proof Alcohol

• Amber or Cobalt Blue Mason Jar w/ lid

• Blender/Food Processor

- Mesh Strainer

- Large Metal Bowl

- Another Large Bowl (Metal or Glass)

- Coffee Filters

Steps:

- Decarboxylate 1oz of weed

- Add the weed to your strainer, then put the strainer in the large metal bowl

- Fill the bowl with water until the weed floats, and let it sit for 90 minutes.

- This should help leech out some of the chlorophyll from your bud.

- Pull the strainer from the bowl so the water drains.

• Collect your wet weed into a ball and squeeze the water out with your hands.

• Break up the squeezed weed and add it to your blender.

• Add about 300ml of your alcohol to the blender and blend on low for 5 minutes.

• Let the mixture sit for an hour, then blend again for 5 minutes.

• Pour the mixture through the strainer making sure to collect the used weed material.

• Make sure to squeeze any tincture out of the material.

• The mixture you just filtered is a potent cannabis tincture! Put it to the side so you can store it later.

• Put the used weed material in a container with fresh alcohol to soak for another hour.

• Pour the mixture through a strainer again, but this time you can discard the used weed.

• Pour your tincture through a coffee filter over a bowl to filter out the tiny particulates.

• This step isn't necessary, but it looks nicer.

• Pour your tincture into an amber or cobalt blue jar that can be sealed.

• Your tincture is ready!

Water Bath Method

The water bath method is a fast way to make tinctures, but it also requires the most care since you have to make sure the water bath doesn't get too hot.

Oddly enough, this method is the lower-budget version of using a Magical Butter Machine since it does all the same things but needs you to be there to take action and monitor for safety.

Important: Do not perform this method with any open flames anywhere in your house! Evaporating alcohol creates a flammable vapor, and having an open flame anywhere near flammable vapor is a recipe for firey disaster. Please be safe!

Supplies:

• Weed

• High-Proof Alcohol

• Mason jar (for cooking)

• Amber or Cobalt Blue Mason Jar w/ lid (for storage)

• Coffee Grinder/Food Processor

• Mesh Strainer

• Large Metal Bowl

• Coffee Filters

• A pot for cooking (not for smoking)

• An accurate candy thermometer or another cooking thermometer

Steps:

• Decarboxylate 1oz of weed.

• Grind up your cannabis.

• Add the weed to your mason jar.

• Add about 300ml of your alcohol of choice to the jar.

• DO NOT CLOSE OR SEAL THE JAR!

• Fill the pot with 1" of water and place on an electric stove (no gas stoves!) on medium.

• Use your thermometer to make sure the water is no hotter than 165°F.

• Place the unsealed mason jar with your weed and alcohol into the pot.

• This is called a water bath. See the picture below to see what it looks like.

• Adjust the temperature as needed until the alcohol/weed mixture gets to 165°F and let it cook for 30 minutes.

• Stay next to the water bath and make sure it doesn't get too hot (above 165°F).

• Remove the jar from the water bath and let it cool for about 30 minutes.

• Pour your tincture through a coffee filter over a bowl to filter out the tiny particulates.

• This step isn't necessary, but it looks nicer.

• Pour your tincture into an amber or cobalt blue jar that can be sealed.

• You're done!

Watch the temperature closely when using a water bath.

Making Tinctures with a Magical Butter Machine

The Magical Butter Machine is the way to make tinctures. It stirs it more, it constantly heats the material, and it has infinite patience, unlike a human being. It can stir and heat your tincture for 8 straight hours with no work on your part past the initial setup.

Supplies:

• Weed

• High-Proof Alcohol

• Magical Butter Machine

• Amber or Cobalt Blue Mason Jar w/ lid (for storage)

• Mesh Strainer

• Large Metal Bowl

• Coffee Filters

Steps:

• Decarboxylate 1oz of weed.

• Add the weed to your Magical Butter Machine without grinding it.

• Add 2cups (or more for a less potent product) of your alcohol to the machine.

• 2cups is the bare minimum you can add.

- Set the temperature to 130°F.

- Set the timer to 4 hours (tincture)

- ...or set it to 8 hours for a stronger product.

- Let the machine finish, then unplug it and let your mixture cool for 30 minutes.

- Pour your tincture through a coffee filter over a bowl to filter out the tiny particulates.

- This step isn't necessary, but it looks nicer.

- Pour your tincture into an amber or cobalt blue jar that can be sealed.

- Tincture time!

Cannabis Tincture with Coconut Oil

Although tinctures can be made with other oils, coconut oil has enough fatty acids to perfectly bind with the cannabinoids. This recipe is somewhat complicated, but you don't need to decarb the weed first.

You'll require:

• Saucepan

• Coffee filters or cheesecloth

• Mason jar

• Grinder

• One cup of coconut oil

• 3 g (0,12 oz) of cannabis

• Glass container

Grind your cannabis first, but skip the decarbing process.

Directions:

1. Pour the weed and coconut oil into a saucepan and place it on a pan. Set it to medium heat for the next 6 to 8 hours. You can also add a little bit of water if you determine that it's needed.

2. After that, just pour the oil into a container, and keep your tincture in the fridge.

Cannabis Tincture with Glycerin

You might ask yourself, is glycerine safe for human consumption? Vegetable glycerine is most likely a part of your diet and you probably don't even know about it, and it's usually ingested through cooking oils.

For this recipe you'll need:

• A mason jar

• 7 g (0,25 oz) or 14 g (0,5 oz) of weed

• 470 ml (2 cups) of organic glycerine

• Grinder

• Hand towels

• Pot

• Coffee filters or cheesecloth

Directions:

1. Grind the weed into small pieces, then perform the decarboxylation. Mix the weed and glycerine in a jar and close the lid. Make sure that all of the plant material is completely covered with glycerine.

2. Line the bottom of your pot with a small towel, and fill it halfway with warm water. The towel will prevent the bottom of the jar from getting overheated.

3. Place the jar in a pot and cook it on low heat for 24 hours. Keep a very close eye on the pot, and shake the jar occasionally.

4. Remove the jar from the pot, let it cool down for about an hour, before filtering the contents of the jar with a cheesecloth.

5. Pour the mixture into a smaller container, and you're ready to enjoy your tincture!

HOW TO COOK WITH CANNABIS TINCTURES

The world of cannabis edibles is continually expanding, and there is no shortage of cannabis companies creating delicious edibles. But did you know that some of the best cannabis-infused foods and beverages can come right out of your own kitchen? While cooking with cannabis oils and butter has been the go-to method for cooking canna-infused food, tinctures are gaining popularity in the cannabis kitchen. In this article, we'll go over the basics of cooking with cannabis and dive into how to use tinctures in your culinary adventures.

The Basics of Cooking with Cannabis

To cook with cannabis, you must use a cannabis product that has been decarboxylated. If you ingest flower as-is, you won't get the effect you are looking for. Why? Because the process of decarboxylation is what activates the cannabinoids in cannabis.

If you're smoking, vaping, or dabbing, the heat you put to the product does the job for you. But if you are cooking, you need to use a product that's already been decarboxylated. Things like cannabutter and canna-oil have gone through the process of decarboxylation, and tinctures are created with cannabis that has been decarboxylated. That's why you can successfully cook with any of these products.

Now that you understand the basics let's focus on cooking with cannabis tinctures.

What's so great about making CBD edibles, anyway?

CBD edibles are great alternatives to THC-based edibles because they can offer relaxation and pain relief without the intense high that is often felt with smoking marijuana or eating THC-based food.

Cannabidiol edibles make the ideal alternative for those who don't want to smoke, who can't smoke, or who find normal marijuana-based products too strong. Edibles also tend to have a more gradual onset but last longer.

CBD edibles can make up a healthy part of your regular diet as CBD oil is rich in Omega-3 oils and amino acids. Edibles are also a great option for people with food restrictions or even those who are just plain picky when it comes to food.

Making CBD edibles is a fun way to experiment in the kitchen. When you have a bit of time and the right ingredients, it's a rewarding way to spend a couple of hours.

Cooking with Cannabis Tinctures

So, what do you need to know about cannabis tinctures when it comes to cooking? Cannabis tinctures are created with a different process than cannabis oil or butter. Canna-oils and butter are created by extracting the cannabinoids into a fat. Because cannabinoids like THC are fat-soluble, these types of products have a high bioavailability, and you'll absorb a large amount of the cannabinoids.

Tinctures, on the other hand, are extracted into high-grade alcohol. This makes them an ideal choice for things like infused candy recipes like THC gummies or lollipops.

Tinctures are also a popular choice for THC infused beverages.

Benefits of Cooking with Cannabis Tinctures

The biggest benefit of cooking with cannabis tinctures is simplicity. You can add them to just about any food or drink, which isn't the case with cannabis oils or butter. I mean, who wants greasy candy and cocktails, right? You can add a tincture to anything you'd like, including juices, soups, ice cream, salad dressing, and even mashed potatoes and gravy. They give you the freedom to be as creative as you want to be!

Another added benefit of cooking with tinctures is precision. With a tincture, you can measure out the exact amount of THC down to the droplet. This is a much more difficult feat with canna-butter.

Other Things to Consider

Remember that ingesting a tincture will work differently than using it sublingually (under the tough). When you use a tincture sublingually, it will absorb straight into your bloodstream within about 15 minutes. When you eat a tincture, it has to pass through your digestive tract where the cannabinoids have to pass through your liver.

Because of the longer process, the onset could take anywhere from 1 to 2 hours. You'll also lose a little bit of potency from ingesting a tincture rather than using it sublingually. That means the number of drops you put under your tongue will have different effects than when you add them to food. But with a little experimentation, you'll find your sweet spot for cooking with tinctures.

WHAT TO LOOK FOR WHEN BUYING A CBD TINCTURE

Now, let's talk about the ten crucial factors to pay attention to when going tincture shopping, whether it be in person or online.

FACTOR #1: LAB REPORTS

A company should provide lab reports on their website to prove their legitimacy and quality, as this has become the industry standard. These lab reports come from a third-party testing facility, which means that the information contained within them is completely unbiased, objective and factual. Lab reports break down everything from the purity level of the hemp to the chemical compounds that it contains. This is not just for CBD tinctures, but for all products.

FACTOR #2: POSITIVE REVIEWS

It's also wise to search for positive reviews on the product you intend to purchase before buying. This way, you'll know the quality of the product, as well as what different customers are finding that it can do for them. Look for reviews both on the company's website and elsewhere.

FACTOR #3: BRAND TRANSPARENCY

One thing that's crucial is that CBD brands are transparent with customers. Due to a lack of regulations in the industry as we all await FDA approval, companies must go above and beyond to tell their customers how they produce their products. Companies that try to hide information from consumers are worthy of your suspicion, so be aware.

FACTOR #4: CORRECT MILLIGRAM STRENGTH OF YOUR CBD TINCTURE

A lot of your potential for CBD success has to do with the milligram strength of the CBD tincture you've selected. For those who don't know, the milligram strength refers to the potency level. How many milligrams of actual hemp extract are within the product's formula directly determines how much CBD and other plant compounds you're taking in per dose. Everyone's ideal milligram strength is unique, as factors like body weight and severity of symptoms all play a role.

Most users experiment with different potency levels before finding the one that's right for them, but look at the range that's available to get an idea of what's a moderate amount, a low amount and a high amount, and choose your ideal strength according to your needs.

FACTOR #5: YOUR PREFERRED TYPE OF HEMP EXTRACT IN YOUR CBD TINCTURE

There are three types of hemp extracts out there: full spectrum, broad spectrum and CBD isolate. Full spectrum contains the complete array of cannabinoids, terpenes and flavonoids that exist in the plant. Broad spectrum is a THC-free alternative that still contains CBD and a limited amount of other minor cannabinoids. Then, CBD isolate is just CBD without any other hemp compounds present.

Each type of extract can give you a unique experience, so make sure that you do some research on how each one can affect you in order to decide which you'd like to try. And, remember that while full spectrum CBD does contain THC, it's only a trace amount, so it can't get you high no matter what.

FACTOR #6: A CLEAN FORMULA

Look at the list of ingredients on the label of the CBD tincture, as companies are not required to adhere to strict rules when it comes to what they put in their CBD tincture formulas. You want to see as few ingredients as possible. Make sure that the non-CBD ingredients that are present are up to your standards and are safe for you to consume.

FACTOR #7: FLAVOR OR NO FLAVOR

Some CBD tinctures are flavored, while others are not. If you have a strong preference, make sure to check whether or not a tincture is flavored before buying it. And, remember that full and broad spectrum hemp tinctures will taste like hemp, so unflavored doesn't always mean flavorless.

FACTOR #8: RIGHT PRICE

We don't want to get ripped off when buying CBD, but CBD tinctures that are extremely cheap may also raise some red flags. Many companies try to prey on naïve first-timers by overcharging, while some brands try to get a competitive edge with super low prices that, at the end of the day, reflect inferior quality. Explore what is on the market to get a good handle on how much a CBD tincture tends to cost, give or take. This way, you'll know if you're paying the right price for a high-quality, legitimate product that can meet your needs.

FACTOR #9: A LONG SHELF LIFE

Something that tends to get overlooked is the shelf life. On average, a CBD tincture lasts for about two years. After that, the chemical compounds start to break down, which means that they lose their effectiveness quickly. This makes the CBD tincture practically useless.

CBD tinctures should have an expiration date on them. When you buy your CBD tincture, make sure that the expiration date isn't coming up too soon, or else you might not be able to enjoy it for as long as you have it in your possession.

FACTOR #10: CO2 EXTRACTION PROCESS

Lastly, we suggest going with a tincture that contains hemp extract produced via the CO2 method. This method is superior, as it results in a cleaner and more chemically stable product.

8 Tips for Using Cannabis Tinctures

The popularity of cannabis tinctures is rising in states where marijuana is legal, and this is understandable, as tinctures were how cannabis was sold in pharmacies across the United States before prohibition of the herb came into effect. Also known as the gold or green dragon, cannabis tinctures are easy-to-make and easy-to-use liquid extracts that are made with alcohol, apple cider vinegar, or vegetable glycerin.

Cannabis tinctures are a great method of consumption for both medical and recreational users who want to avoid smoking or don't like the intensity of ingesting marijuana-infused products. Tinctures are also a good choice for children or adults who want to try cannabis for the first time because they are easy to administer in small doses. If you've chosen to try some for yourself, here we offer eight tips for using cannabis tinctures. Enjoy!

1. The best way to use a cannabis tincture is to take in the drops directly under your tongue, as this absorbs the mixture directly into your bloodstream for almost instantaneous effects.

2. Disguise the taste of your cannabis tincture by diluting it in a little juice or water flavored with honey (never for to a child under one year of age), a slice of ginger, or fruit.

3. Avoiding eating or drinking for at least 15 minutes after taking your cannabis tincture for the best results.

4. Add your cannabis tincture to meals and drinks like sauces, smoothies, salad dressings, soups, and sherberts as an alternative to taking a dose under your tongue.

5. Add 1-2 droppers full of your cannabis tincture to an 8 oz. Cup of warm water to make an instant tea.

6. To give a tincture to a baby, the mother or woman nursing the baby should take it as the therapeutic compounds will pass through the breastmilk.

7. Take great care to keep the mouth of the glass dropper for your cannabis tincture clean to avoid impurities contaminating the batch with mold. Don't ever touch it to your mouth, your bare hands, or an unsterilized surface.

8. Store your cannabis tinctures in a cool, dark, and dry place, and they will last you for years.